Toe the Line

HOW I CONQUERED INGROWN TOENAILS

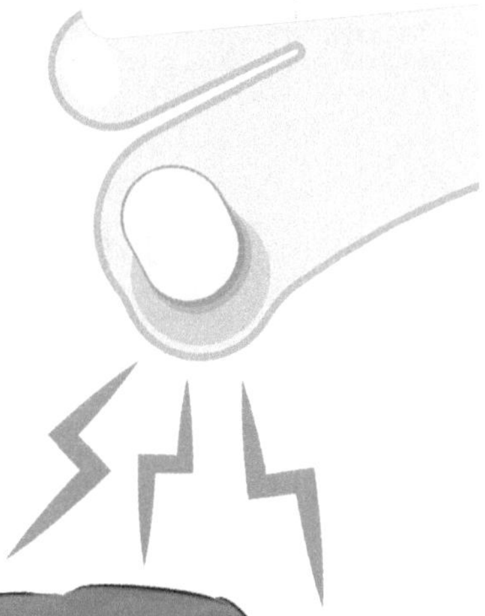

PERSONAL EXPERIENCE WITHOUT ANY SURGERY

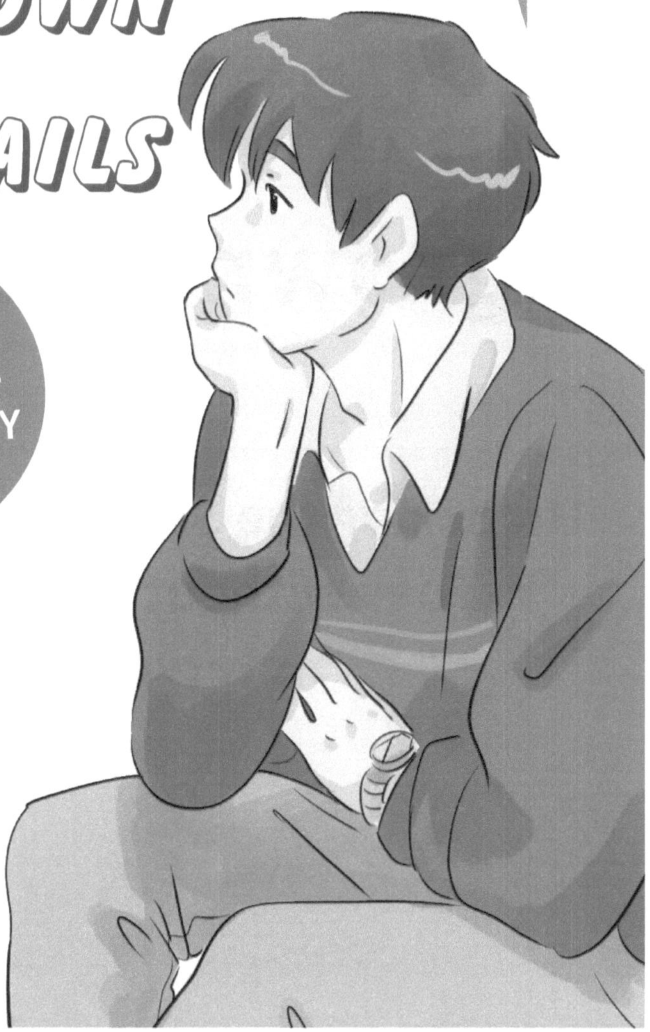

Guide to Navigating Toenail Troubles

by Tanmay

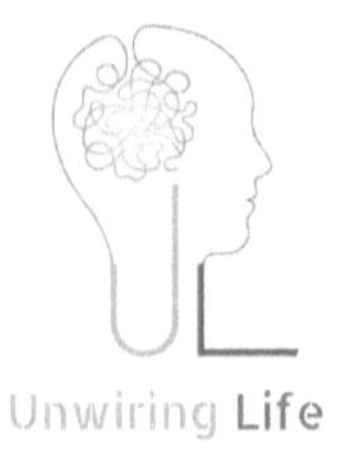

Toe the Line

How I

Conquered

Ingrown Toe nails

Unlocking the Secrets to Pain-Free Toes Without Any Surgical Intervention

i

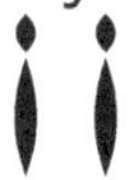

About The Author: Tanmay

Hey there, I'm **Tanmay**! Trust me, I know just how excruciating an ingrown toenail can be—it's like your toe's worst nightmare, right?
Well, I've had that nightmare three times over, and each time I learned something valuable. Even after two surgeries, the problem persisted, and it was both frustrating and disheartening. That's when I stumbled upon a simple yet effective home remedy that not only worked wonders for me but also for my friends and family.

Disclaimer: Although I can't guarantee this will work for everyone—I'm not a medical professional, after all—I genuinely believe in its effectiveness. Always consult your healthcare provider for medical advice tailored to your individual needs.

To me, one's mindset is the ultimate game-changer. Harnessing the power of my subconscious mind helped me stay resilient throughout this journey. And here's the kicker—if you **follow this procedure** as diligently as I did, there's a good chance it will work for you too.

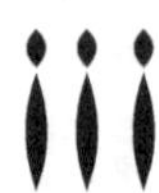

Navigating This eBook

Toe Topic 1: Introduction

The Day Badminton Wasn't Fun Anymore

I've always been a badminton enthusiast, rallying early morning birdies with my friends at the local park. Dressed in my modest $25 sports shoes, I thought I was fully geared up for my daily games. All seemed well, except for a nagging pain in my toe, which I brushed off as a minor irritation. But one day, I just couldn't ignore it anymore.

The Unpleasant Surprise

That fateful day, when I returned home and removed my shoes, I felt something wet on my toe. To my shock, it was leaking pus. The pain was excruciating. My trip to the doctor confirmed my worst fear: I had an ingrown toenail, and I might need surgery.

The Dilemma: To Cut or Not To Cut

Surgery seemed like an extreme measure for what began as an annoyance during my badminton sessions. I started to question, is going under the knife the only way out? This was a question that needed an answer, not just for me but for millions out there suffering the same agony.

Charting the Unknown Path

So, here we are. In this eBook, I'll walk you through my journey, from the initial days of discomfort to finding an alternative way out of this painful predicament. We'll explore the common causes, the conventional medical solutions, and the less invasive home remedies that I experimented with.

It's All in the Mind

While the physical aspect was challenging, the mindset was equally crucial. I came to understand that your mental frame plays an essential role in dealing with any life obstacle, not just an ingrown toenail.

Ready, Set, Go!

If you're reading this, chances are, you're also grappling with this pesky issue. So, come along as we navigate this together, toeing the line between conventional wisdom and innovative solutions.

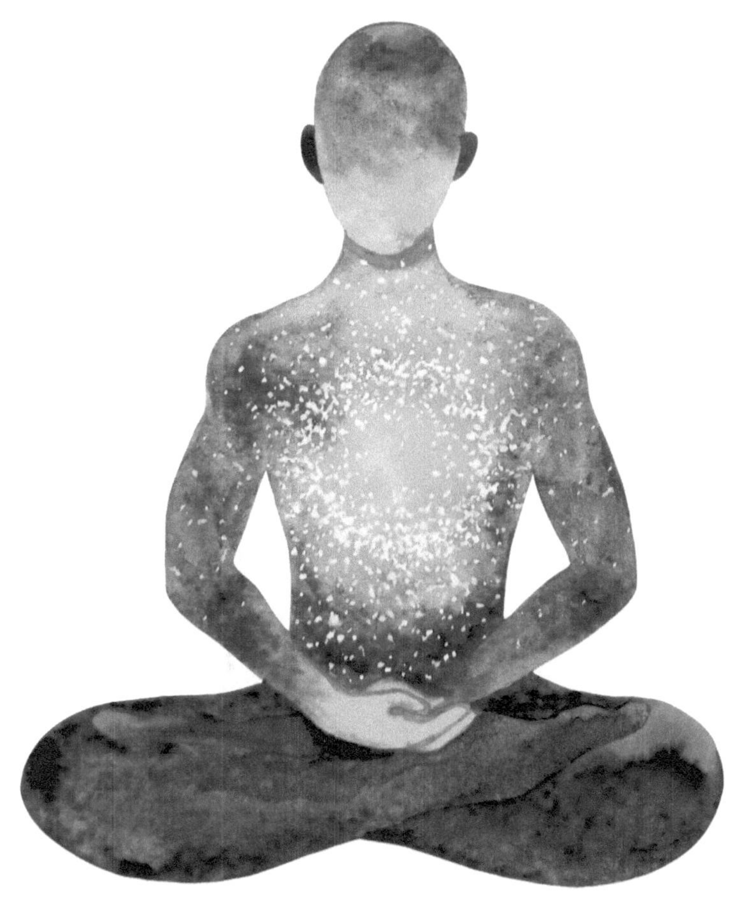

Toe Topic 2: What Are Ingrown Toenails?

The Scientific Explanation

Before we dive deep into the nitty-gritty, let's understand what we're up against. In medical terminology, an ingrown toenail, or onychocryptosis, is a condition where the edge of the toenail grows into the flesh surrounding it. This leads to symptoms like redness, swelling, and in severe cases, infection that results in pus formation.

The Reality Behind the Pain

While the medical explanation seems quite technical, the reality is much simpler but painful. The nail curls inward and starts to dig into your skin. Just imagine a small, sharp knife slowly penetrating your flesh. Ouch, right?

Not Just A "Toe" Problem

Don't be fooled; an ingrown toenail isn't just a toe problem. It can significantly affect your daily activities. Think about it; your toe is part of almost every movement you make. Walking, running, or even standing becomes a herculean task.

The Age Factor

While it's common to assume that this issue predominantly affects the elderly or those with specific medical conditions like diabetes, the truth is, it can happen to anyone, at any age. Yes, even those in their twenties who enjoy a good game of badminton can fall victim.

The Pain Spectrum

The severity of the pain can vary. Some days, it's just a minor annoyance that you can ignore. But there will be days when the pain is unbearable, and even a soft touch can send shivers down your spine.

<u>Toe Topic 3: Common Causes</u>

The Usual Suspects

Ingrown toenails are not random events that happen without rhyme or reason. There are several common causes that lead to this painful condition. These include:

Wearing the Wrong Footwear

As mentioned in my personal story, wearing cheap or ill-fitting shoes can significantly contribute to the problem. Such footwear can compress your toes, leading to a variety of issues, including ingrown toenails.

Incorrect Nail Trimming

This is something many people are guilty of. Cutting your toenails too short or not in a straight line can encourage the nail to grow into the surrounding skin.

Trauma to the Toe

Physical injury, whether from stubbing your toe against a door or engaging in high-impact sports, can also be a leading cause of ingrown toenails.

Genetic Tendency

For some, the issue might be genetic. If your family has a history of ingrown toenails, you may be at higher risk.

Other Medical Conditions

Other health issues like diabetes or fungal infections can also make you more susceptible. Poor circulation, particularly in the lower limbs, can worsen the condition.

Summing It Up

Understanding these common triggers can not only help you treat your current ingrown toenail but also help prevent future occurrences. In the following sections, we will explore how to tackle these issues effectively.

Toe Topic 4: Traditional Medical Solutions

The Go-To Solutions: Are They Really Solving the Problem?

When it comes to dealing with ingrown toenails, the first instinct is often to visit a doctor for medical advice. But let's take a closer look at these conventional treatments, many of which I've personally tried without long-term success.

Prescription Medication: A Temporary Fix

Doctors often prescribe antibiotics for infections and topical creams for inflammation. But let me tell you, these are often just band-aid solutions that don't get to the root of the problem.

Surgical Procedures: A Painful Cycle

I've been through the drill — from partial nail removal to more invasive surgeries. The procedures were not just expensive but also incredibly painful. And the worst part? The problem usually recurs.

Podiatrist: The High-Cost Specialist

Consulting a podiatrist might seem like the ultimate solution, but let's not forget how costly these specialist services can be. Not to mention, the issue often comes back after treatment, putting you back at square one.

Over-the-Counter Treatments: The Mirage

Antiseptics and bandages might seem like an easy fix, but from personal experience, they don't offer a lasting solution.

What's Often Overlooked: The Real Issues

Traditional treatments usually ignore crucial lifestyle factors, such as the type of footwear you choose or how you trim your nails, which can prevent the issue from returning.

The Harsh Reality

All these conventional methods do is drain your wallet and test your pain threshold, without offering a permanent solution. I found myself caught in a cycle of temporary relief followed by recurring agony.

The Limitations of Conventional Treatment

Having been through the medical route with its endless cycles of antibiotics and painkillers, I realized that something was missing. These solutions were not only expensive but temporary. The question then was: Is there a better way?

A Nod to Ancient Wisdom

Often dismissed as myths or old wives' tales, traditional methods of healing have a wealth of wisdom to offer. These are remedies passed down through generations and have stood the test of time.

Mind Over Matter: The Real Game-Changer

One of the most powerful tools in our healing arsenal is our mindset. It's not just about applying a remedy; it's about truly believing in its potential. Our subconscious mind plays a massive role in how effective any treatment can be.

Affordability and Accessibility

Why break the bank with expensive treatments when you can have a cost-effective solution right in your kitchen? It's not just about saving money; it's about taking control of your own health.

A Holistic Approach to Healing

Home remedies offer more than just symptomatic relief; they aim to treat the root cause of the problem. When coupled with the right mindset, they can offer a comprehensive solution that benefits your overall well-being.

Beyond the Recipe: Testimonials

It's not just my story; many have found relief and a better quality of life through home remedies and a strong mindset.

The Journey Ahead

Are you ready to break free from the limitations of traditional medical treatments? Are you prepared to harness the power of your subconscious mind and natural remedies?

Toe Topic 6: My Journey with Home Remedies?

Hitting the Breaking Point

There's a limit to how much pain and discomfort you can endure before you say "enough is enough." I had reached that point. Frustrated with the cycle of antibiotics and temporary relief, I decided to seek a different route.

The First Step: A Natural Alternative

My 82-year-old grandfather, a wise man with a deep respect for Ayurvedic practices, suggested a natural remedy that he'd been using for years. Skeptical yet desperate, I decided to give it a shot. The result? Let's just say the persistent pain began to ease after only a few applications of this Ayurvedic marvel.

The Role of the Subconscious Mind

I firmly believe that it wasn't just the ancient Ayurvedic wisdom that eased my pain. It was my mindset, my conviction that a natural solution could work. My subconscious mind seemed to align with my conscious efforts, bolstering the entire healing process.

Trial and Error: Crafting the Perfect Remedy

Miracles don't happen overnight. I went through rounds of trial and error, experimenting not just with natural ingredients but also various mind-calming techniques. And then, after weeks of tweaks and persistence, I landed on a regimen that did wonders for me.

Going Beyond Myself: The Bigger Picture

I couldn't keep this revelation all to myself. I started sharing it with my inner circle—friends and family struggling with similar issues. The impact was universally positive. It dawned on me that my story had the potential to alleviate the suffering of others.

How Shocking Were The Results?

So groundbreaking that it led me to write this eBook. I didn't just regain my ability to move, play, and live without constant pain; I reclaimed my life. All of this was made possible not just by a simple remedy, but also by the right mindset and the specific technique on how to apply the remedy effectively. This synergy between belief, method, and natural ingredients opened up a new chapter of wellness for me.

Feeling this transformative change compelled me to help others. I know firsthand how debilitating the pain can be, and I don't want anyone else to go through that ordeal if they don't have to.

If you're grateful for the insights this eBook has provided and want to say thank you, the best way you can do that is by spreading the word. Tell at least three people about this eBook and ask them to continue the chain by informing three more people.

<u>Toe Topic 7: Step-by-Step Guide to My Home Remedy</u>

The Ultimate Guide to Conquering Toe Pain: An Ayurvedic Approach with Proven Results

Why Believe in This Method?

If you're rolling your eyes at the mention of Ayurveda, hold on. This isn't any run-of-the-mill solution; it's backed by a **4.3+ star rating** on Amazon and priced at approximately **$2** for a **100ml bottle** . But remember, the magic isn't just in the magical oil. It's in how you use it. Follow the steps outlined below, accompanied by visual aids, for optimal results.

NOTE: You can easily get this life saviour Ayurvedic oil, from Amazon. If Amazon doesn't ship to your location, don't sweat it!

Reach out to me directly on Telegram at **<u>unwiringlife</u>**, and I'll arrange something for you.
Additional shipping and tax costs will apply for international orders.

Ingredients

The secret sauce in our method is an Ayurvedic oil, which I'll reveal later in the guide. It's what makes the entire procedure effective and fast-acting.

- Cotton
- Purified water
- A ladle
- Paper Tape, scissor
- Polythene bag
- MAGICAL AYURVEDA OIL- **"NOORANI TEL"**

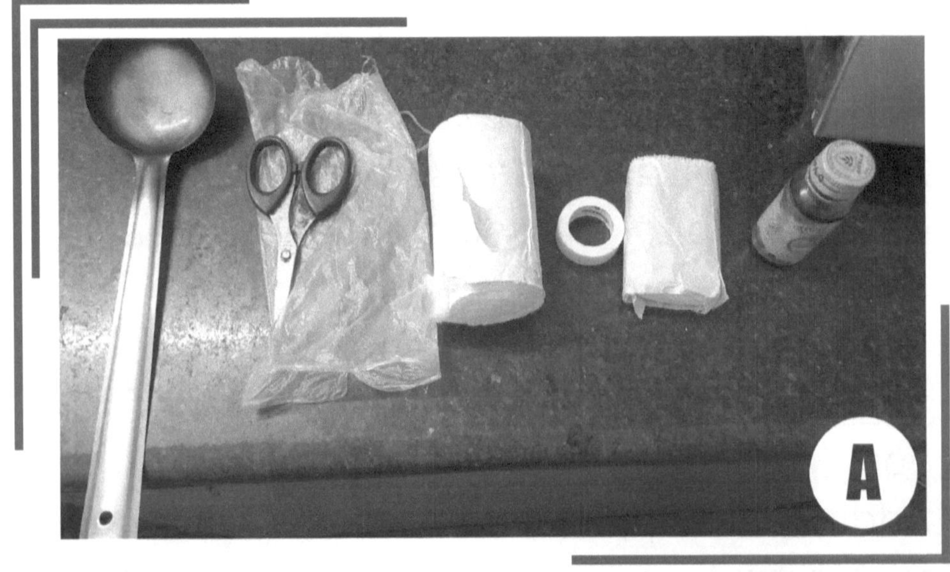

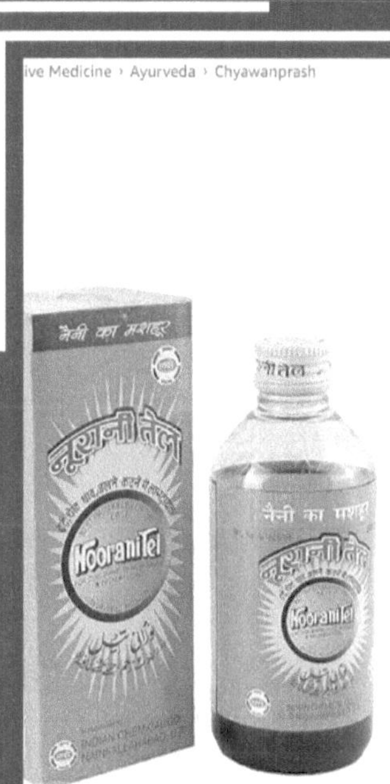

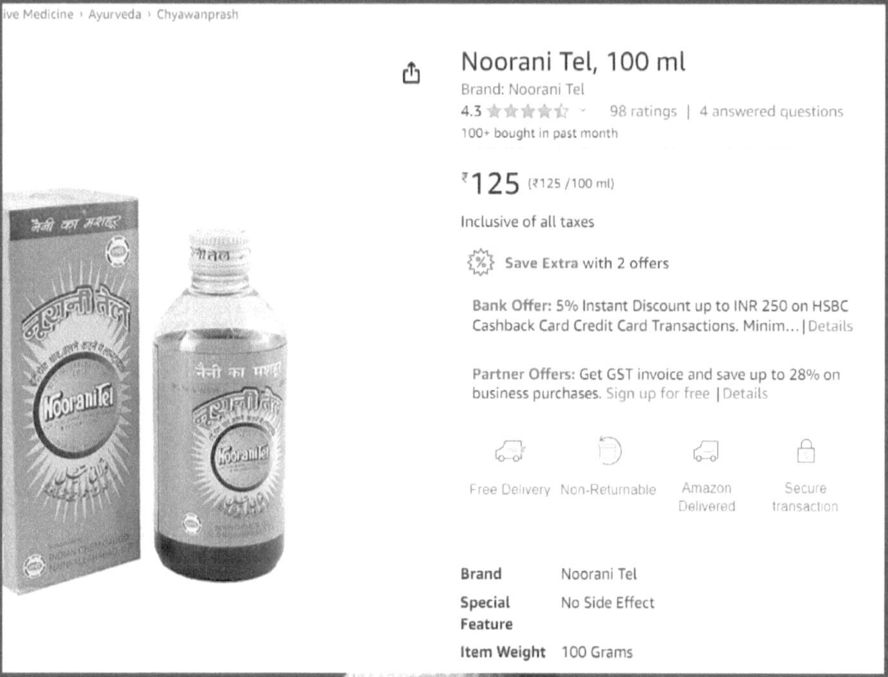
ive Medicine › Ayurveda › Chyawanprash
Noorani Tel, 100 ml
Brand: Noorani Tel
4.3
98 ratings | 4 answered questions
100+ bought in past month
₹125 (₹125 /100 ml)
Inclusive of all taxes
Save Extra with 2 offers
Bank Offer: 5% Instant Discount up to INR 250 on HSBC Cashback Card Credit Card Transactions. Minim... | Details
Partner Offers: Get GST invoice and save up to 28% on business purchases. Sign up for free | Details
Free Delivery
Non-Returnable
Amazon Delivered
Secure transaction
Brand
Noorani Tel
Special Feature
No Side Effect
Item Weight
100 Grams
NooraniTel

50 ml
नूरानी तेल
BEST PAIN KILLER OF THE EAST
NooraniTel
FOR CUTS BURNS PAINS WOUNDS & INFLAMMATIONS
UNANI MEDICINE
INDIAN CHEMICAL CO. MAUNATH BHANJAN U.P.

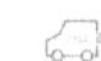

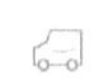

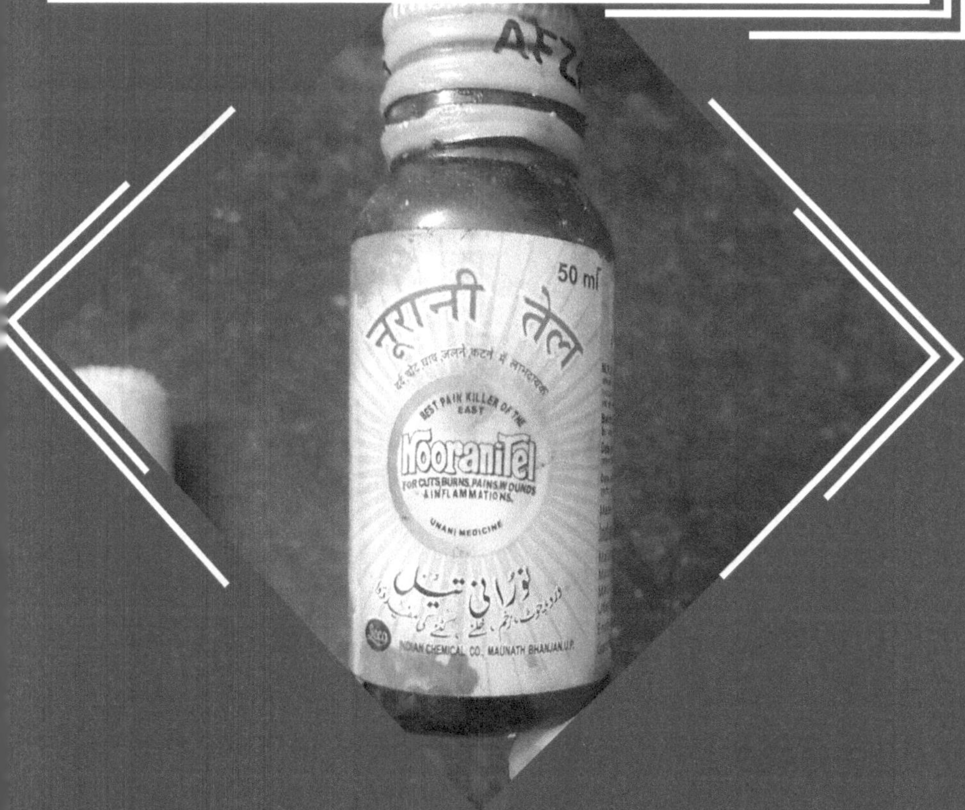

- <u>On Amazon.in</u>, the item is priced at approximately ₹125, which is around $2 at most.

- However, the same item costs around $52 on <u>Amazon.com</u>.

If you're unable to find it on Amazon or find it too expensive, feel free to reach out to me on Telegram at @**<u>unwiringlife</u>**.

I can purchase the item from the local market in India and ship it to you. While I can't provide an exact cost at this moment, as it would depend on your location and shipping charges, I estimate the total cost to be between $20 and $40, which is likely cheaper than purchasing from Amazon.com.

I'll update you with the precise details before shipping. Just let me know if you're interested!

<u>Here's the Amazon link for your convenience</u>

Please note: Carry out the procedure that I'm about to explain on the next page. Do this 1-2 hours before you go to sleep and keep the bandage on for the next 24 hours for optimal results. Do it for X days + 7 extra days, [X days = untill your pain get vanished.]

<u>If you have any doubts or issues, you can message me on my telegram username-</u>

@unwiringlife

The Application Method: It's More Than Just The Oil

Step 1: Prepping the Cotton

Take a piece of cotton and roll it into a small disc that can easily roll up. Soak this cotton disc in RO or purified water—remember, tap water can have impurities that may cause irritation. Make sure the cotton is wet but not dripping. Squeeze out any excess water, refer image, b,c , d, e, f.

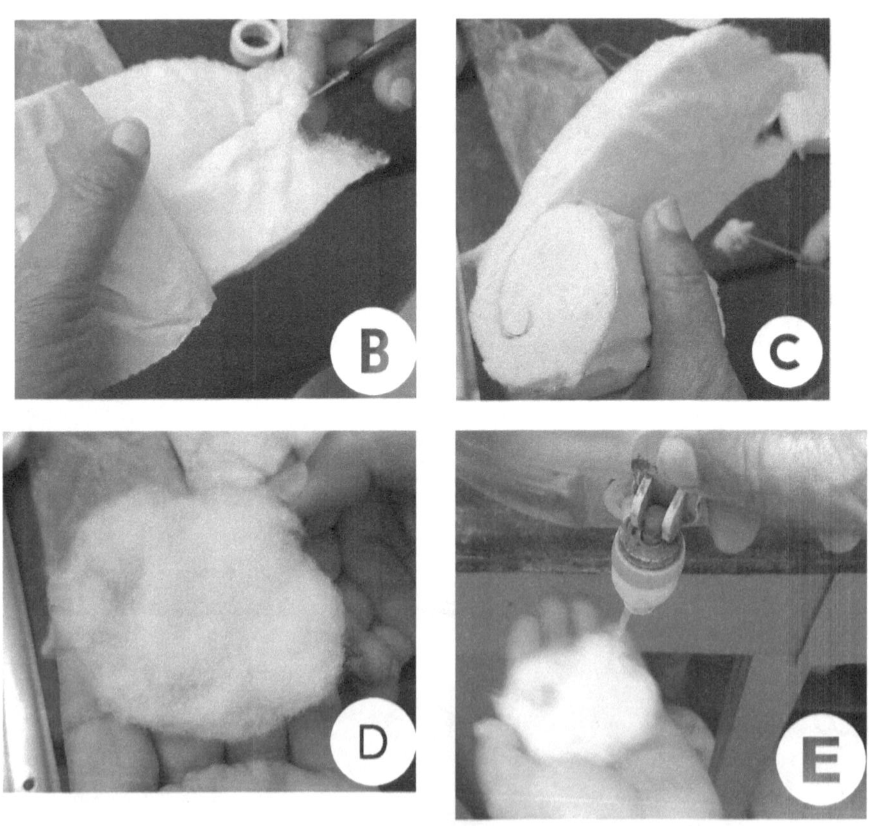

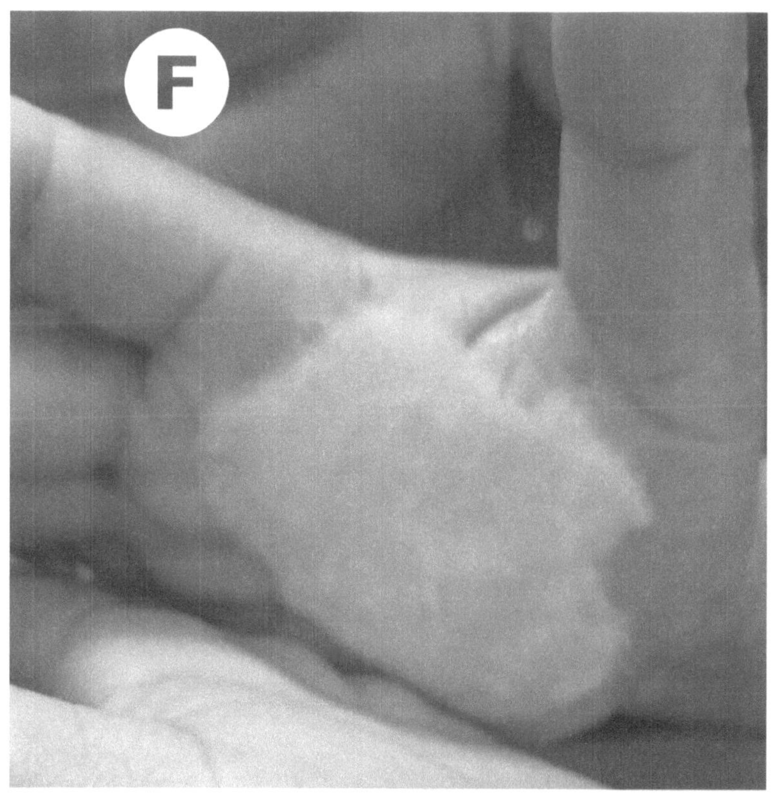

Step 2: Heat That Oil Up!

Unscrew the bottle cap off your Noorani Tel. Take a full spoon of the oil and pour it into a ladle. Place the ladle over a low flame until it's hot but not smoking—nobody wants a fire hazard! Once it starts to vaporize, it's ready, do not burn it, if it turned black or catch fire then you have to start the process again. refer image, G,H,I,J,K.

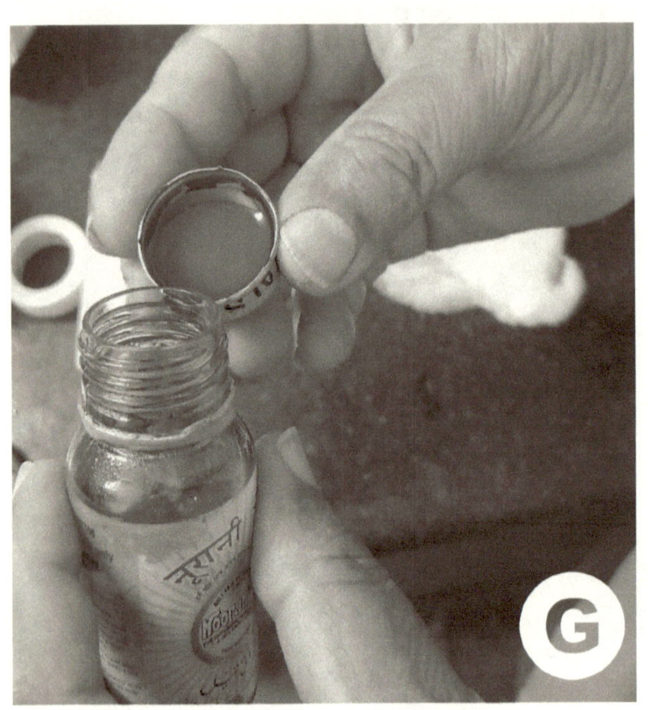
G

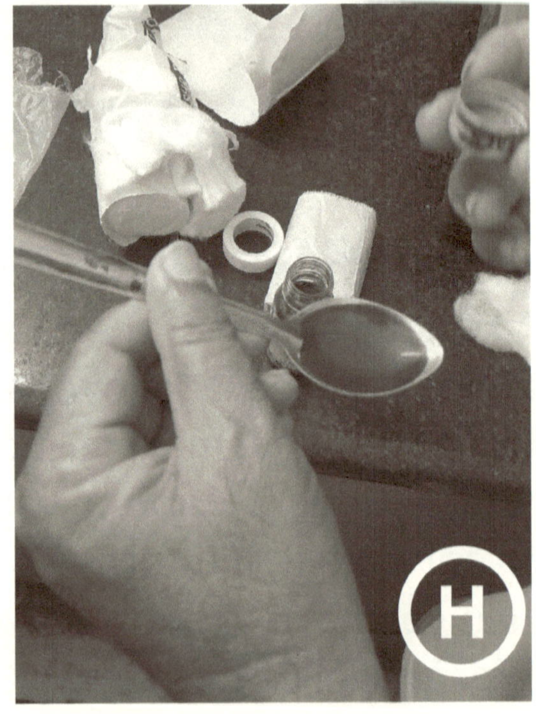
H

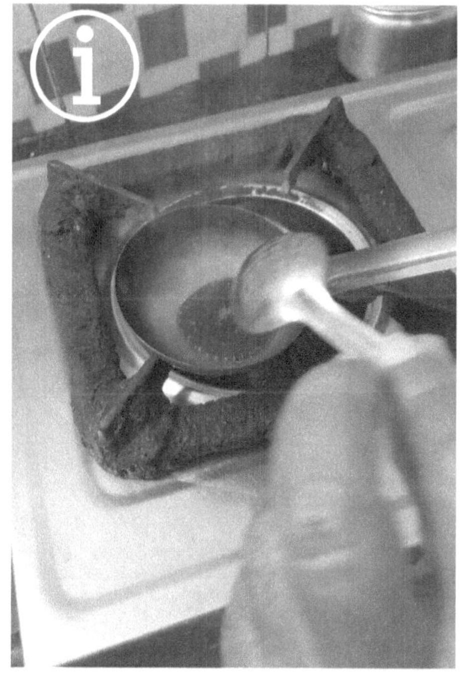

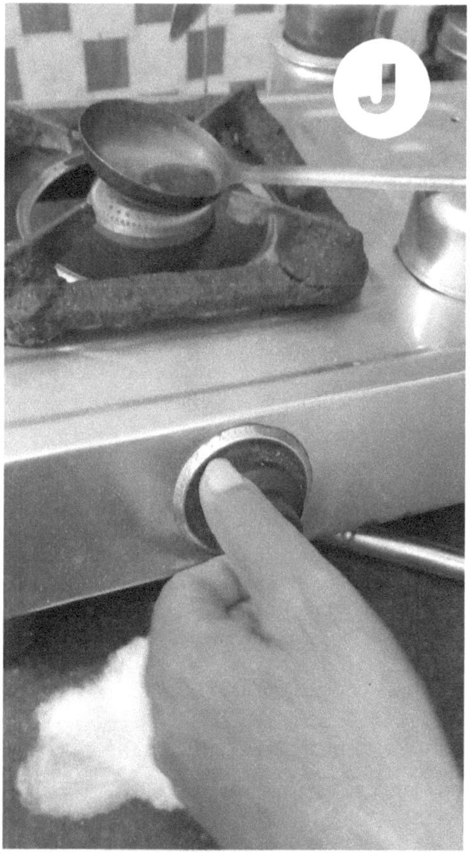

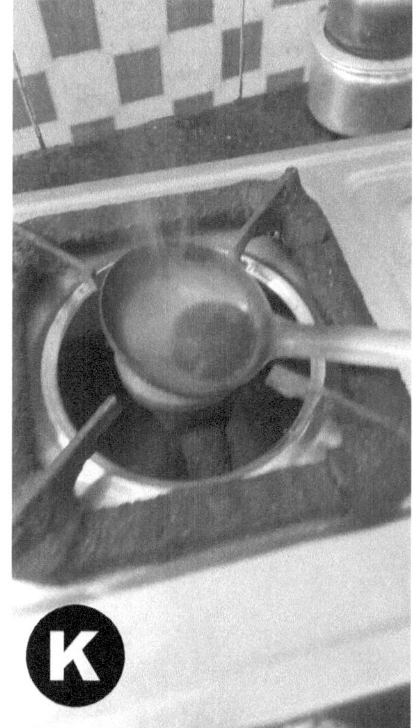

Heat it for few seconds on low flame

Step 3 : Soak the Cotton

Dip the wet cotton disc into the heated oil. The cotton will absorb the oil and turn a shade of red, indicating it's soaked well.

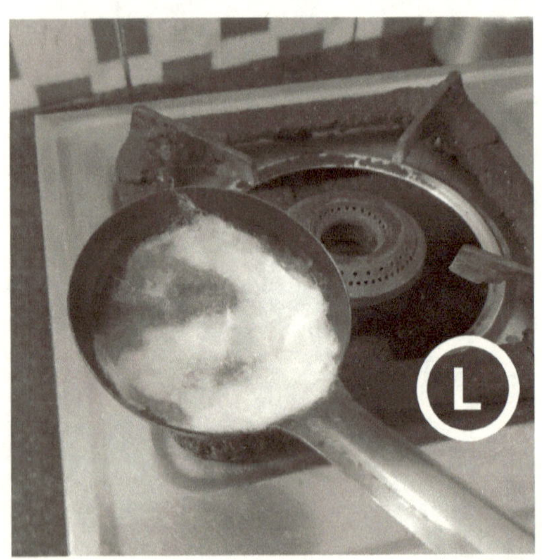

Press with spoon evenly, so that oil spreads on complete cotton

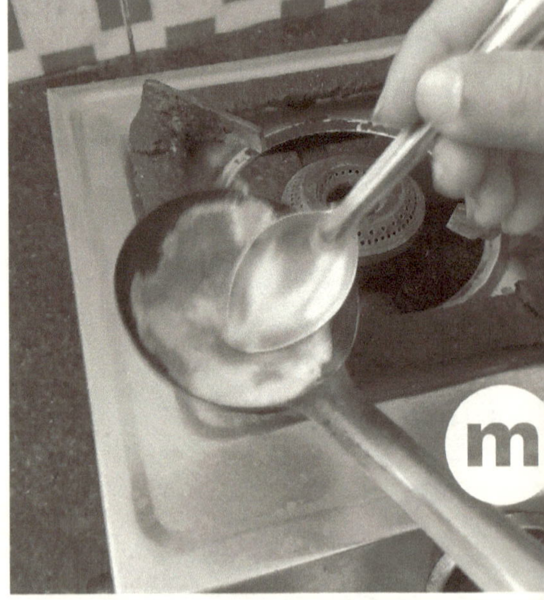

Step 4 : Application Time

Place this red, oil-soaked cotton on the toe where you're experiencing pain. Make sure the oil-soaked cotton is warm, as heat can amplify its healing properties. Carefully place the warm, oil-soaked cotton on the toe where you're experiencing discomfort. Gently press it against the affected area, ensuring good contact with your skin. Hold it there for about a minute.

If you start to feel a burning sensation, remove the cotton and allow your skin to cool for a few seconds. Then reapply the cotton and repeat the process. Continue this cycle of applying and removing the cotton in intervals of 1-2 minutes for maximum effectiveness.

Remember, it's important to follow this method closely—no taking shortcuts!

Refer image - n,o,p

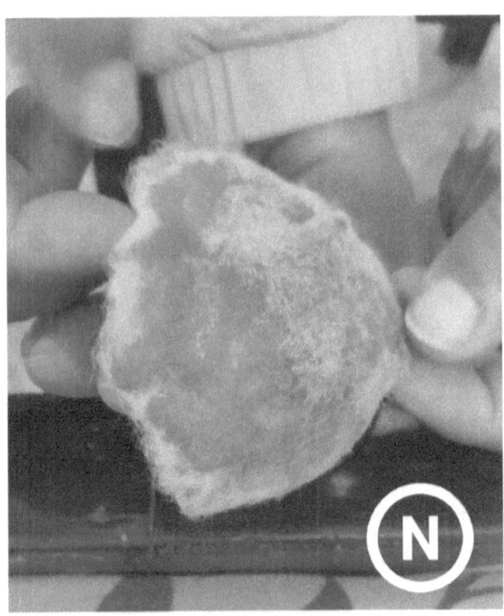

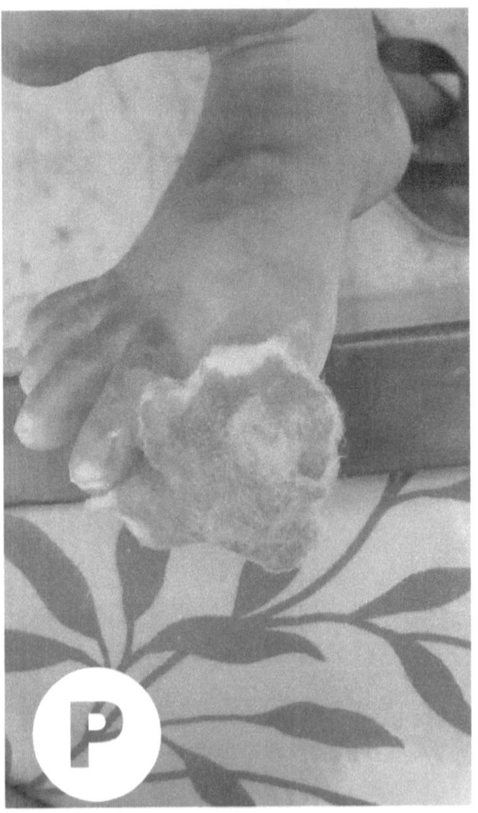

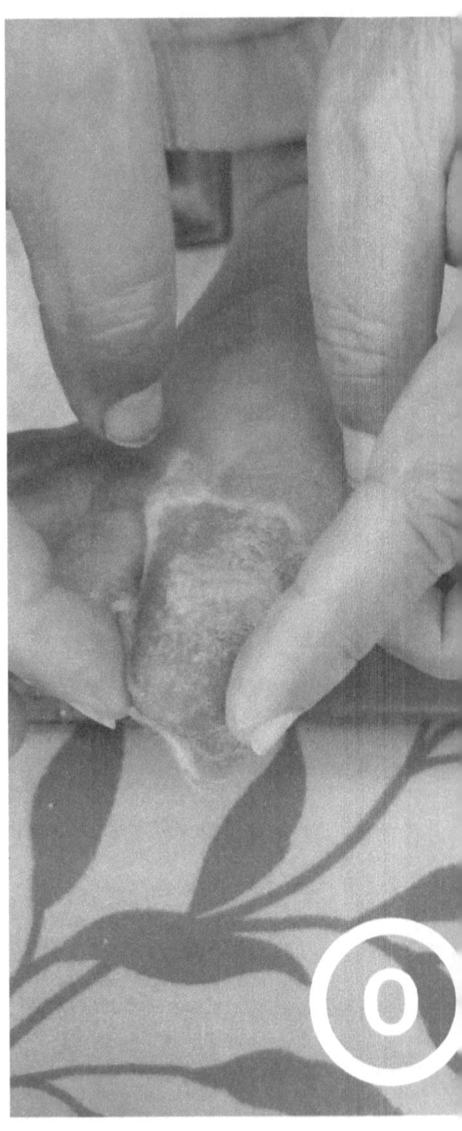

Do fomentation for 1-2 minutes while the compress is still warm.

Step 5: The Wrapping it-Up

Wrap the cotton around your toe, secure it with some white tape, and cover it with a small polythene bag. This ensures no oil leakage throughout the night. This should be done 1-2 hours before you go to sleep.

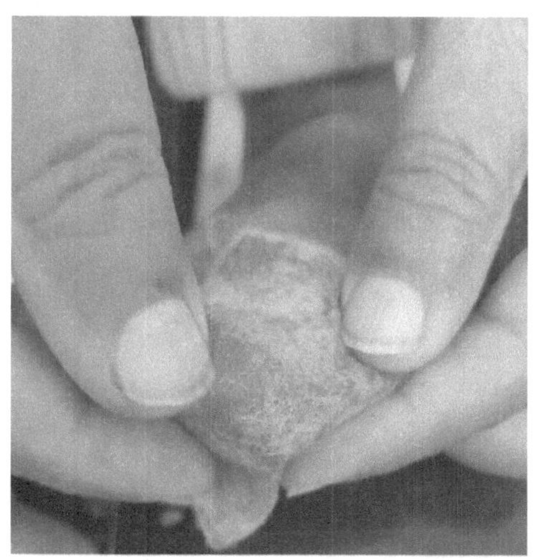

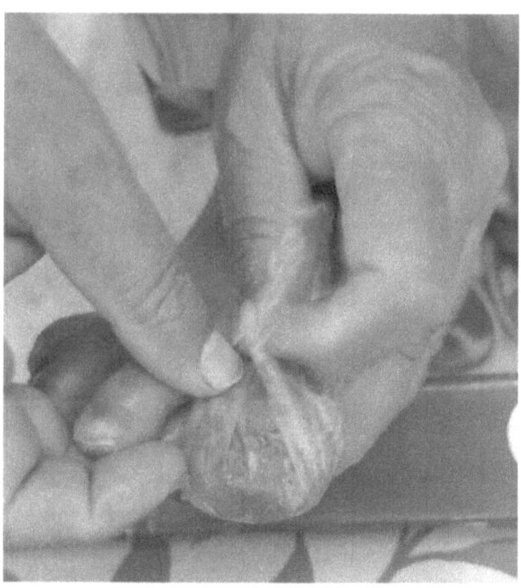

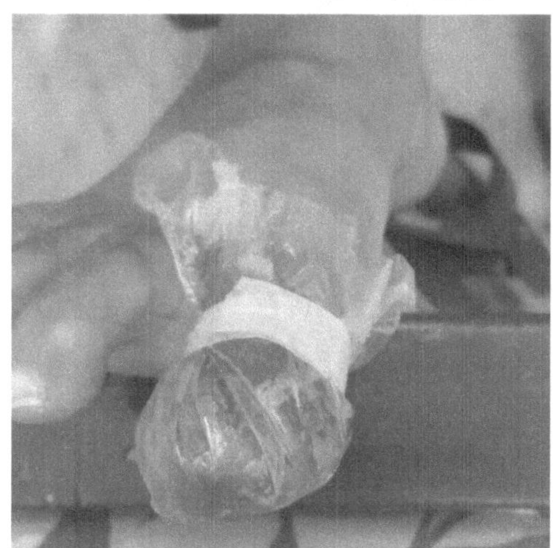

1) Wrap cotton with oil

2) wrap polythene

3)put paper tape

4)then roll the band

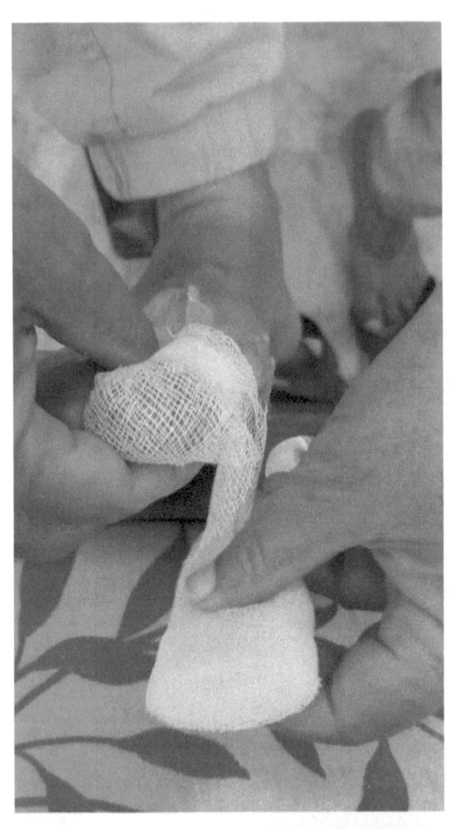
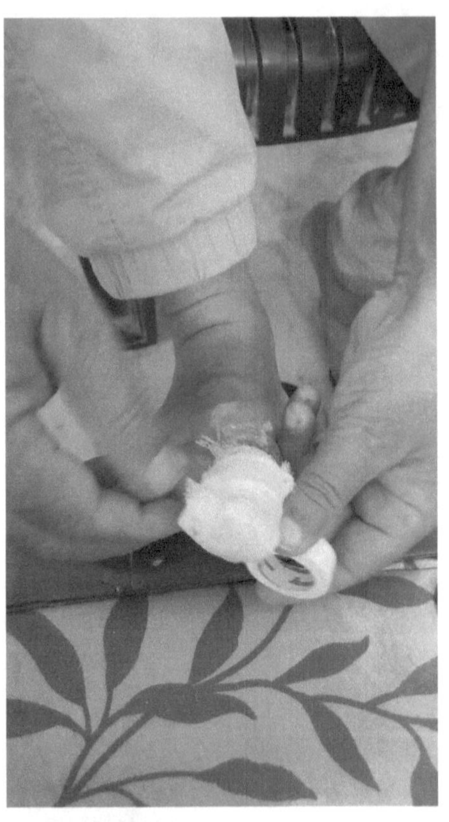
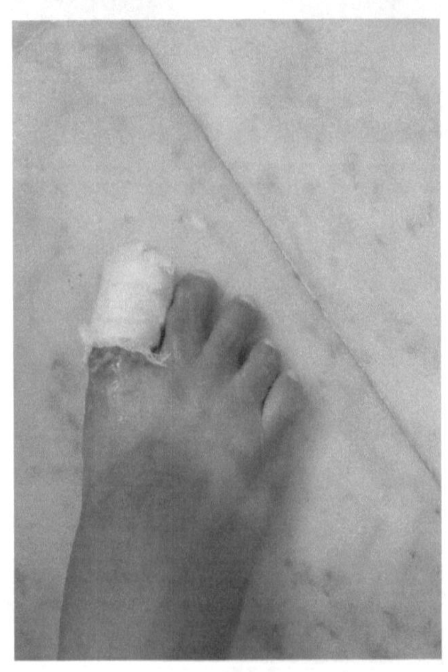

Repeat for 24 Hours

The next day, carefully remove the cotton and dispose of it. Clean the area with fresh cotton soaked in a bit of water. Allow it to air-dry for an hour. Then, start the whole process over for another 24-hour period. Remember do it 1-2 hours before going to sleep.

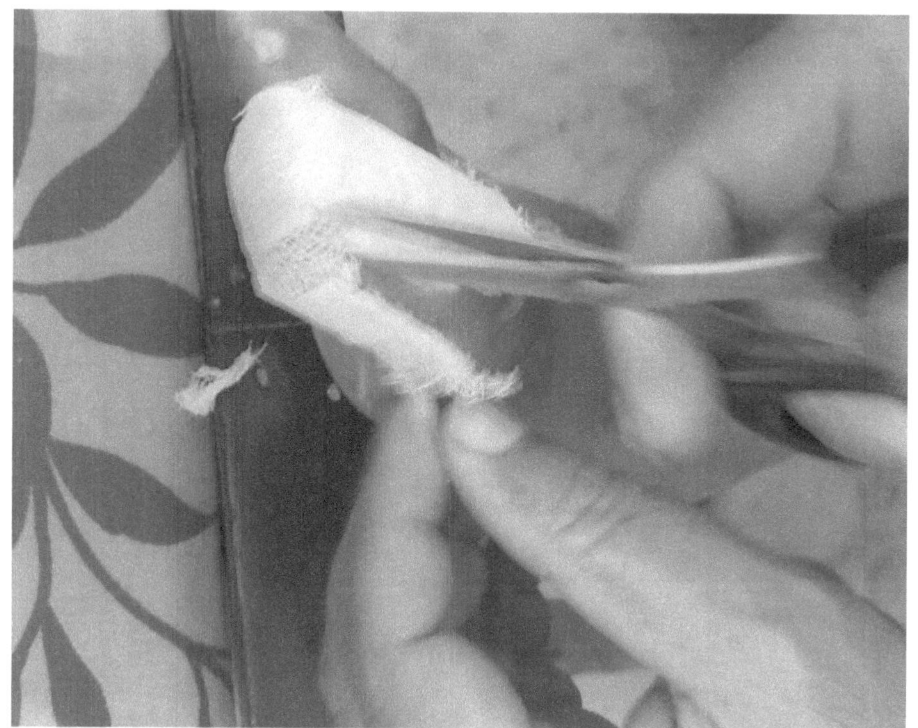

After-Care and Prevention -- Extended Treatment

After you've started feeling relief from the toe pain, you might think that's the end of it. But hold on! Continue the treatment for at least an additional 7 days. This is a crucial step to ensure that the pain doesn't just go away, but stays away.

Variable Timeframe

Understand that the timeframe for this treatment isn't set in stone. Some people might experience relief within 5-6 days, while others might need up to 10 days or more. For example, if it takes you 10 days to completely eliminate the pain, then you should continue this procedure for at least another 7 days. I know it might seem tedious, but it's crucial for complete healing.

Why Extra Days?

You might be wondering, why the extra days? The main reason is that the extended treatment ensures your toe heals completely and it helps prevent future issues. The added time allows your nail to soften and helps to draw out any remaining pus and infection.

Continued Comfort

Congratulations! By this point, your toe pain should be a thing of the past, and you should be able to walk barefoot without any discomfort.

You might even be feeling grateful and thinking about how to thank me—buying me a coffee wouldn't be a bad idea, LOL! ---> https://www.buymeacoffee.com/vichaarit

The Next Important Step: Prevention

Now that you're back to walking like a normal person, the crucial thing is to keep it that way. And the most important factor in preventing a recurrence is your choice of footwear. If you're using tight shoes that irritate your toes, throw them out. Replace them with shoes that are one size bigger than your current size. And it's essential to pick high-quality shoes with a soft form. The inside of the shoe should be gentle enough that even if your toenail makes contact with the wall of the shoe, it doesn't stick but moves along. For example, I find Sketchers incredibly comfortable —no, this isn't sponsored. You can choose any brand, but make sure they are soft and have a spacious toe box

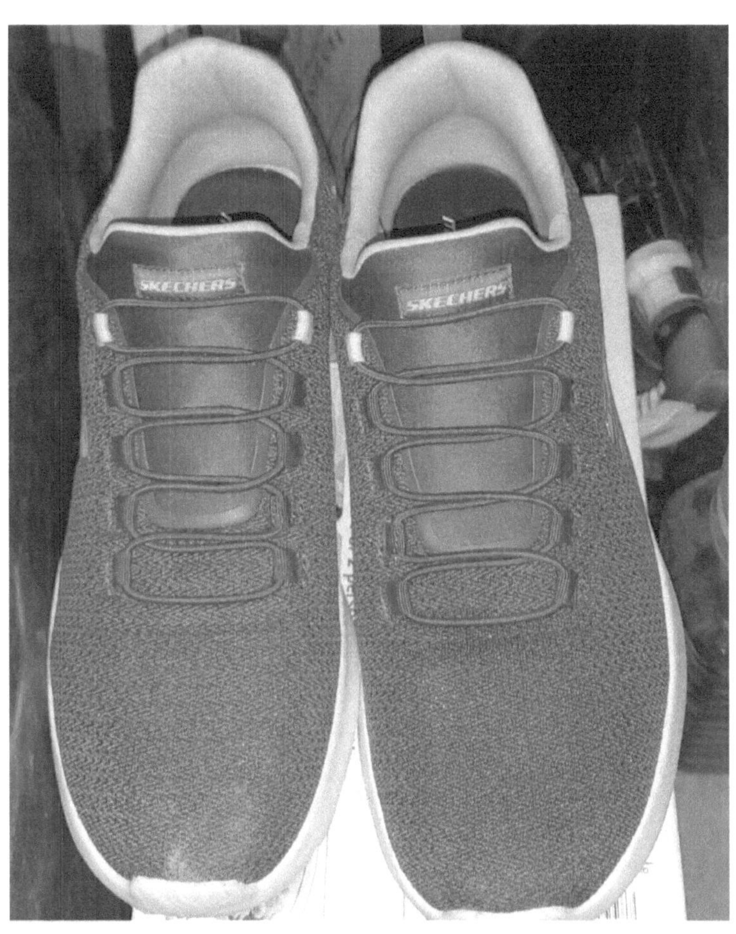

I strongly recommend **not wearing** Clogs, as they are closed at the front and tend to fit loosely. This loose fit can cause your toes to press against the front of the shoe, potentially leading to the development of ingrown toenails.

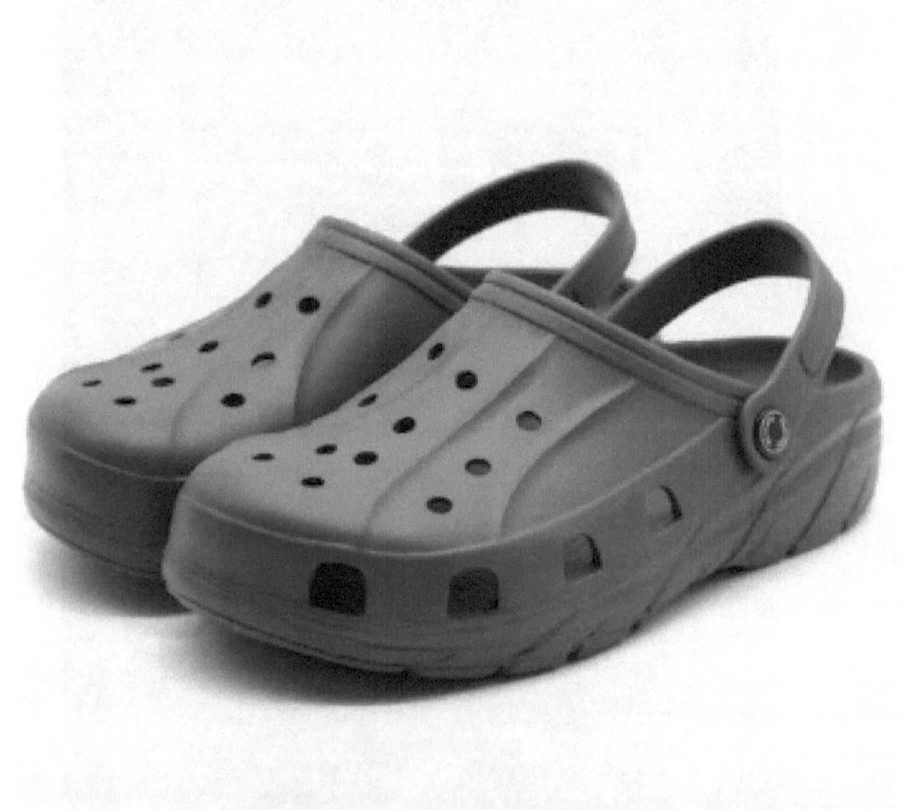

Nail Care Tip for Preventing Future Intoe Nail Grow

One of the most effective ways to prevent future toe pain is to properly maintain your toenails. Forget about using a nail cutter; it can be too harsh and cause ingrown nails.

 Instead, use a nail file to gently grind down the edges of your toenails. Aim to do this at least once in 15 days, following a warm foot soak which softens the nails and makes them easier to file. This simple, yet highly effective, routine can be a game-changer in preventing future bouts of toe pain.

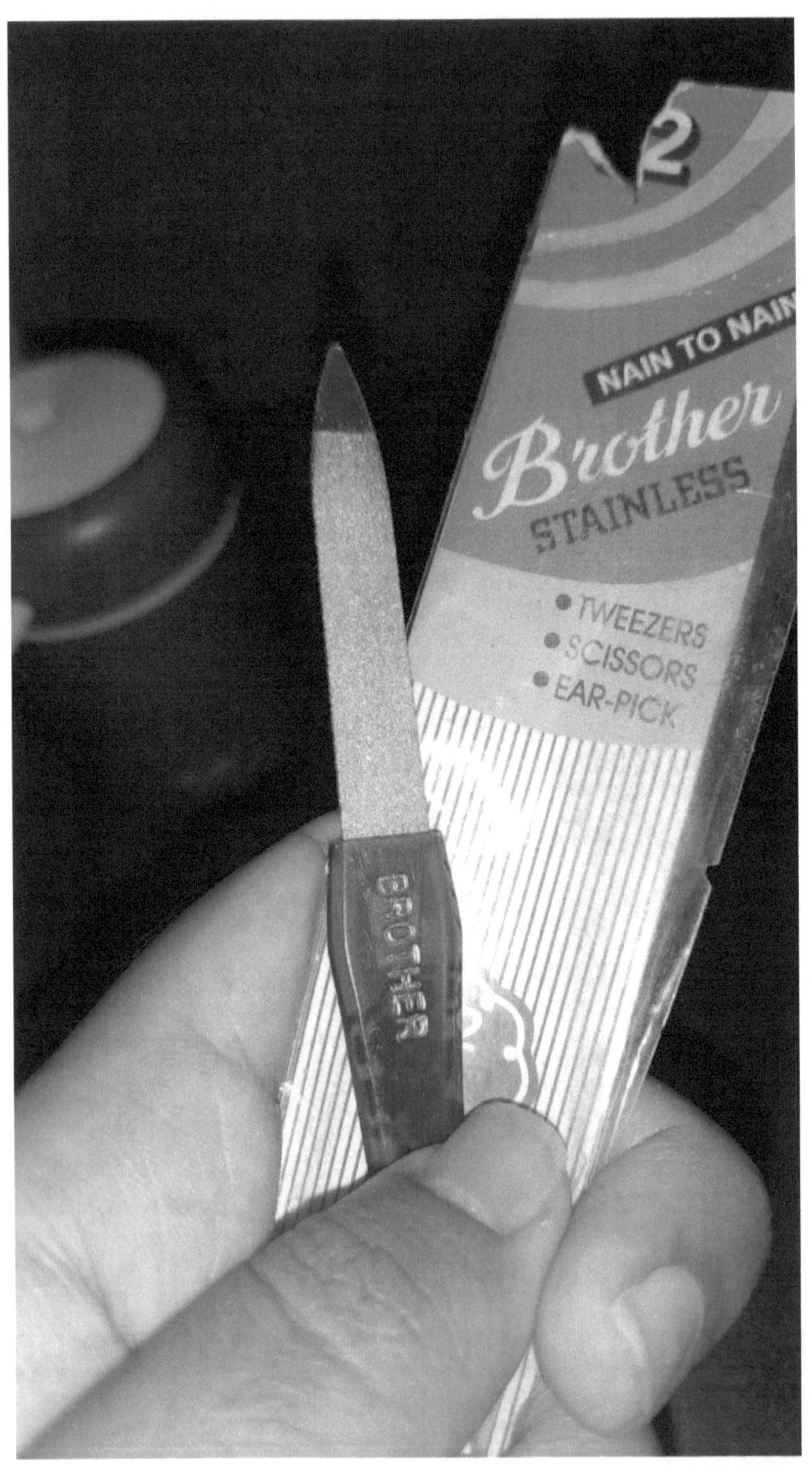
2
NAIN TO NAIN
Brother
STAINLESS
• TWEEZERS
• SCISSORS
• EAR-PICK
BROTHER

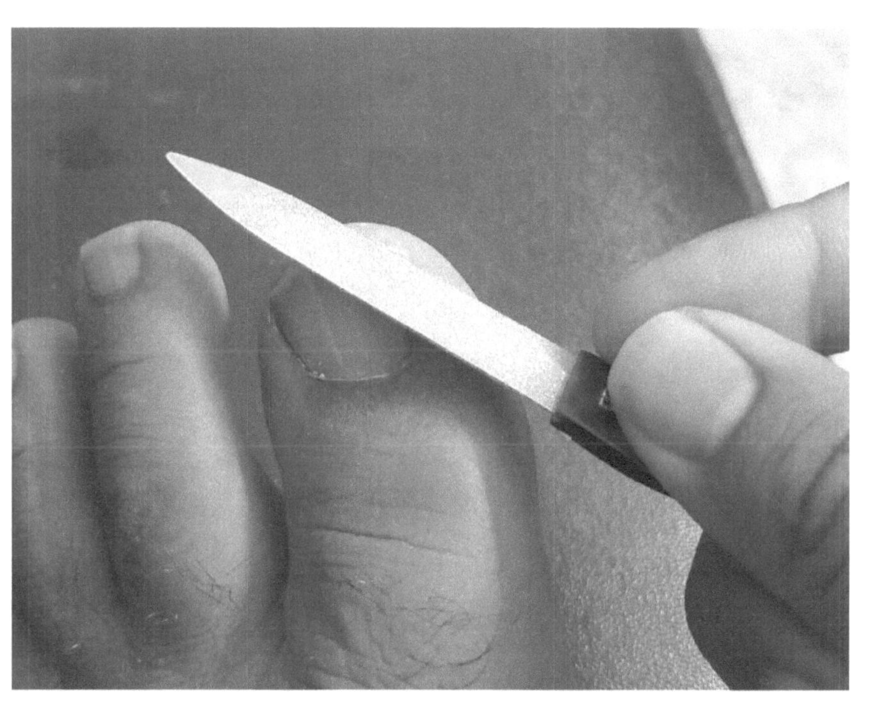

by following this, you will

never have intoe nail grow problem again

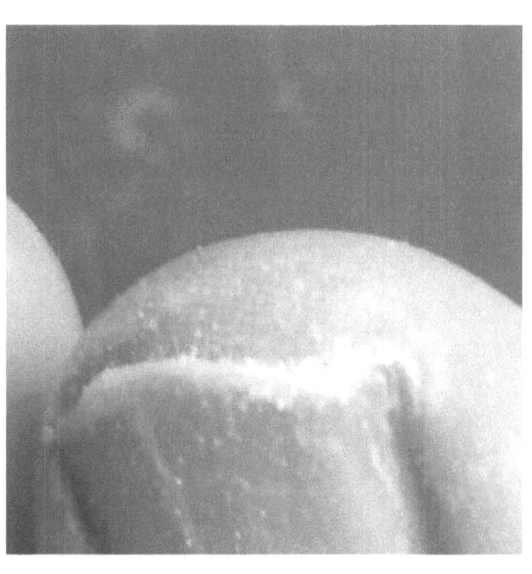

TOE TOPIC 9 - Testimonials

Why Are These Testimonial Pages Blank?

You might be wondering why these pages are empty. Well, to be completely transparent, these blank pages are **waiting for your feedback**.

As of now, I don't have testimonials because this is a newly launched method that I firmly stand by.

 While it has helped me and those in my immediate circle, I didn't want to include fake testimonials just to fill the space—**I want to keep things real**.

How Can You Help?

If this guide helps you conquer your toe pain, I would be incredibly grateful if you could share your experience with me. Send me your feedback on Telegram at **@unwiringlife**. Your testimonial could be featured in the next edition of this eBook or even in a physical book. Let's collaborate in helping others relieve their pain and improve their lives.

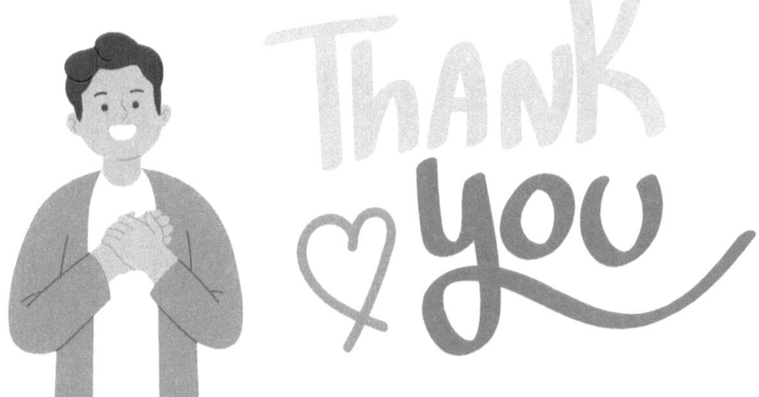

Thank You for Reading!

Firstly, a huge thank you for investing your time and trust in this guide. Your well-being is the primary reason this guide exists, and I hope it serves you well.

Conclusion:

By this point, you should have all the tools you need to not just manage, but conquer your toe pain using an Ayurvedic method that's stood the test of time. This isn't some quick fix or a band-aid solution; it's a lifestyle adaptation aimed at offering you lasting relief and prevention. When followed diligently, this remedy can eradicate your ingrown toenail issue from the root, eliminating the need for surgical intervention altogether. Stick with the routine, be meticulous with after-care, and never underestimate the power of subconscious mind.

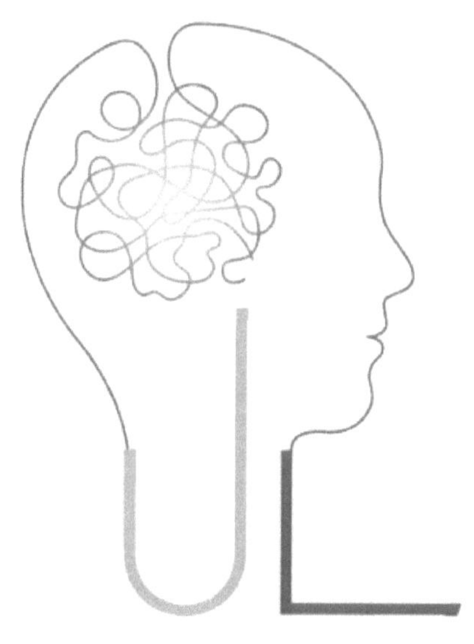

Important Links for Your Journey:

- <u>Noorani Tel on Amazon</u>: If it's available in your region, this is your quickest option.

- <u>Not on Amazon?</u>: No worries! Directly message me on Telegram at unwiringlife for ordering details.

- Buy Me a Coffee: If this guide has helped you, feel free to **BUY ME A COFFEE**

  https://www.buymeacoffee.com/vichaarit

- <u>Send Your Feedback</u>: For testimonials for this eBook, reach out on Telegram at @unwiringapps.

Again, thank you for your time, and I can't wait to hear about your success journey. Your testimonies will not only validate the guide but also help countless others who are in pain. Here's to a pain-free life!

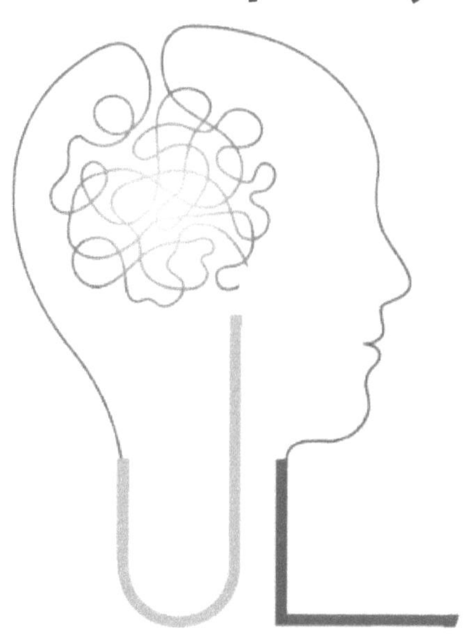

✹ The Ultimate Guide to Conquering Toe Pain ✹

Put an end to the excruciating pain of toe issues. This guide will introduce you to an Ayurvedic approach that targets the root cause, potentially saving you from costly and invasive surgical procedures.

About the Author

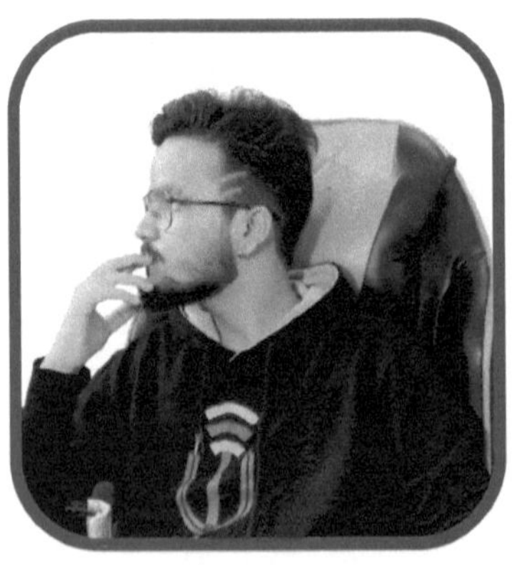

Tanmay Agarwal, the founder of Unwiring Tech and its different sub-brands like Unwiring Apps, Unwiring Life, is on a journey to make a real impact. He's keen on harnessing the incredible power of the subconscious mind to change lives for the better.

For more, check out www.unwiringtech.com

www.unwiringtech.com

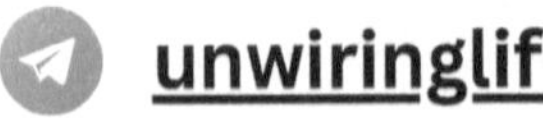 unwiringlife

ISBN 978-93-6013-093-0